Taking another Road

By
Lynne D M Noble

Copyright 2018 Lynne D M Noble

Independently published

Contents

Acknowledgement

I think that, whenever there is a writer in the house, other family members have to learn a few extra rules. These include remembering to keep quiet just when the writer is holding a number of important concepts in their head and putting up with the masses of paper which appear to land on every conceivable space in the house. In fact, it takes a special sort of person to live with a writer.

This acknowledgement recognises the contribution that my husband, Michael, plays in supporting my working environment.

Preface

The definition of pain is that it is a highly unpleasant physical or mental sensation which can be caused by illness, injury or emotional suffering. Some people who are suffering pain may think this is a fairly bald understatement.

There are a few people who do not feel physical pain – congenital analgesia – at all Most of us will experience pain in its many forms as it has a protective role to play. Pain produces a reflexive retraction from harmful stimuli and protects the body while it heals. Pain, for example, limits the use of the area affected by illness or injury, giving it time to heal.

During times of emotional anguish we may withdraw from the fast pace of life and find a quieter place to be which is less hurried. Sometimes we can find solace in music or the beauty of the countryside. We instinctively know what it is we need to do to begin our healing. We also need time to heal when we have a physical ailment but we have forgotten how to do this. Even when we are at deaths door we do not allow ourselves time to recuperate. A couple of 'duvet days' would hasten overall recovery but, in our society, it is frowned upon.

Our instinctive responses to certain types of pain are known as 'guarding.' This helps in limiting use which assists the healing process. Even though people are subconsciously aware of this they have failed to apply it to their own healing.

Pain can be initially divided into two categories. There is acute pain which starts suddenly and is short term. Chronic pain is often defined as any pain which lasts for more than twelve weeks. It may stem from acute pain which is a normal sensation that alerts us to illness or injury but the sensation of discomfort in chronic pain is entirely different. It is often accompanied by decreased appetite, mood changes, fatigue and, sleep disturbance among others.   It may require an entirely different treatment approach than that of acute pain.

Pain is specific to each individual. It affects both the psyche and the body and our reaction to prior pain also affects how we experience it in the future.

When pain receptors are irritated they cause pain. Pain receptors can be found in the joints, skin and internal organs.

Psychogenic pain can occur when there is no obvious damage to tissues.

Nerve pain occurs when the peripheral nerves, brain and spinal cord are damaged. Nerve pain - also known as neuropathic pain - is often described as stabbing and requires different analgesia from nociceptive pain which is the general pain we can sometimes have.

Whatever type of pain we have, the process of pain starts with nerves which send information to the brain. The brain interprets this pain. In effect the pain is not in our body. It is generated in our brain so that the process of pain has far greater complexity than is first realised.

Pain can also be further classified into visceral pain (organs) and somatic/body pain which includes the muscles, bones, skin and joints.

Our experience of pain depends on a number of factors including the strength of the stimulus, the resilience of the individual and individual susceptibility. Our pain receptors are sensitive to

- physical stimuli such as that produced by stubbing your toe, distension of bowel or joints moving beyond their normal range
- thermal stimuli – eating something that is too hot or cold, for example. . The threshold for thermal stimuli ie where sensation becomes actual pain is heat that is above 42C and cold at below -15C.
- and chemical stimuli which are irritants like acids, alkali and irritants

It is good to be able to classify pain. Different painkillers have different actions and may work in the central nervous system or in the peripheral nervous system. Being able to identify the likely cause of pain enables us to prescribe the correct medication for that ailment.

This book is intended to inform about the different types of pain and, just as importantly, what painkillers are most likely to be the optimal response to a specific pain. The book will look at some of the over the counter medications and, some prescription drugs. However, its main intention is to look at effective analgesia which is not mainstream analgesia. Most people have enough knowledge about paracetamol and ibuprofen but do not know about some equally effective compounds which can be used as adjunctive pain relief or as a standalone analgesic and further, often work more quickly and for longer periods and without some of the side effects of commonly prescribed or over the counter medications.

This book, in no way, replaces the knowledge of your GP but is a useful and comprehensive source of knowledge for those who wish to further their knowledge of pain.

Acute and Chronic Pain

Be patient and tough; someday this pain will be useful to you
Ovid

To begin to understand pain - and which treatment is best for a specific pain - there are a number of concepts which need to be understood. The first of these is understanding the difference between acute and chronic pain.

Acute pain is caused by the activation of pain receptors throughout the body from stimuli. The pain is not diffuse – which can happen with chronic pain. The location of acute pain is instantly known and it is caused by tissue damage. It has a set purpose – that of alerting you to the injury and protecting you from further injury.

With chronic pain, the reason for the pain may not be known; there may be no known prior illness or injury yet chronic pain continues and may vary in intensity without any apparent cause. Alternatively, an injury may have healed yet the pain continues. Sometimes chronic pain occurs as a result of unresolved inflammation. For example, rheumatoid arthritis is one such condition. It may also occur due to damage to the nervous system as in neuropathic pain (traumatic injury, stroke and post-herpetic neuralgia and multiple sclerosis) and unknown precipitating factors such as is seen in Fibromyalgia.

While acute pain is short lived, chronic pain is seen as pain which continues for longer than twelve weeks. It appears to serve no adaptive purpose.

How do we feel pain?
Acute pain

- A harmful substance is detected by receptors that are situated on the cell membrane of the sensory nerve ending found in organs and in the skin.

- The receptors are proteins. They are made in the cell body and then transferred to the surface of the nerve ending.

- Different receptors determine the type of stimulus that the nerve cell can respond to.

- Pain stimulates pain receptors

- The stimulus is transferred via specialised nerves to the spinal cord and then to the brain.

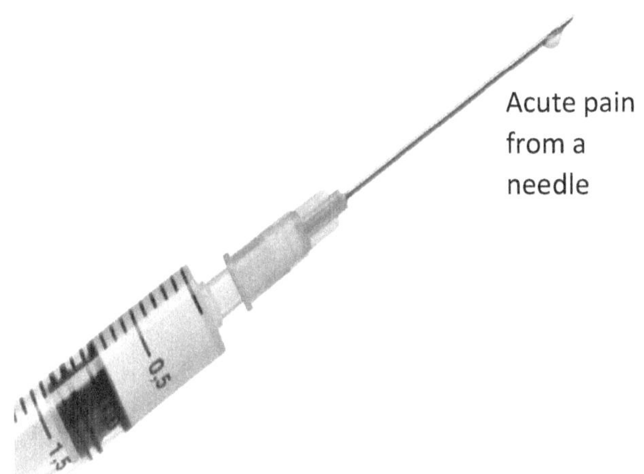

Acute pain from a needle

Chronic pain is pain which lasts for longer than twelve weeks. It is more of a dull, thudding background pain in contrast to acute pain, which is sharp and sudden. There are more medications which act on chronic pain that can usefully address acute pain. With chronic pain there is often no obvious injury and the underlying cause is entirely different from that of acute pain.

The activation of microglia which are cells in the central nervous system are responsible for chronic pain [1] Microglia are the macrophages (scavengers) of the central nervous system. Studies have shown that spinal microglia were activated in response to injury of peripheral nerves.

When minocycline (an antibiotic which can cross the blood brain barrier) was administered to rats it was found to prevent pain. Minocycline inhibits microglia and other cells such as astrocytes from

---

[1] theconversation.com/what-causes-chronic-pain-microglia-might-be-to-blame-6173

'cross talking' with neurons. It has been firmly established that this cross talk is necessary for the development of chronic pain.

It was thought that microglia only participated in the development of neuropathic pain but recent studies show that microglia activation[2] also contribute to the maintenance of chronic pain.

Summary

Acute pain is short-lived and is felt through pain receptors on the end of sensory nerves. It helps prevent further injury.

Chronic pain is any pain which continues after 12 weeks. There may be no apparent illness or injury.

---

[2] Microglial activation is understood as a change in cell number, morphology, phenotype and motility, the expression of membrane-bound and intracellular signaling proteins, and the release of immunoregulatory products, such as cytokines and chemokines. Microglia express a range of receptors that detect ligands released as a consequence of neuronal injury, and that lead to their activation

Microglia are implicated in the development and maintenance of chronic pain. It does not help prevent further injury occurring.

Other types of Pain

As well as acute and chronic pain, we can place pain into further categories.

Breakthrough pain is pain which occurs between the administrations of regular scheduled painkillers. In some cases the dose of painkiller can be increased but in some cases this is not possible without being harmful. Some people may turn to alternative medicine to alleviate breakthrough pain. This may include aromatherapy, acupuncture or massage. Many amino acids have powerful anti-inflammatory and analgesic properties. They can be used alongside prescribed and over the counter medications as an adjunctive medicine although they can just as easily be used as the primary medication. The therapeutic value of amino acids will be discussed in more detail later in this book.

Soft tissue pain occurs when organs. Muscles or tissues or damaged and inflamed. They are generally amenable to paracetamol and NSAID's, cold compresses for the first couple of days and then alternating heat and cold after that. Elevating the affected part and resting are essential for rapid healing. The Acronym RICE

- Rest
- Ice
- Compression
- Elevation

Is still as true today as it has always been. Of course, where anti-inflammatories cannot be taken then alternative anti-inflammatories should be considered since soft tissue pain is often reluctant to resolve and can often move into the realms of chronic pain.

Nerve Pain is not ameliorated by using over the counter painkillers. Neuropathic pain occurs due to damage to the nerve and are generally amenable to medications which treat depression and epilepsy.

Antidepressants work by increasing the body's own pain fighting resources. They do this by inhibiting pain signalling at the level of the spinal cord. That is, they dampen pain signals.

The medication for neuropathic pain cannot generally be obtained over the counter and many – such as amitriptyline have side effects including sleepiness and long standing brain fog. Magnesium is an alternative solution (please see section on Magnesium).

Referred Pain is pain when pain from one part of the body is felt in another. Pain from gallstones may be felt radiating from front to back. Pain from kidney trouble may be felt around the shoulder blade. Referred pain requires a little detective work in order that the appropriate treatment is given.

Phantom Pain occurs when there is pain in the part of the body which has been removed. Some patients may feel pain in their leg even after it has been amputated.

This occurs because whenever an injury occurs, pain is registered in the brain and creates a physical neurological pathway. Even after a limb is amputated the pathway is still there with its potential for feeling pain.

On a smaller scale, all pain as a result of injury will create a neurological pathway where it is registered. This will become more entrenched the longer an injury remains unhealed. It is therefore of great importance that pain is addressed as soon as is possible. The stoic among us, who do not resort to painkillers, may be troubled with long standing pain as a result of the neurological pathways which have 'captured' the pain resulting from the injury.

Total pain includes the emotional, social and spiritual factors that affects a person's pain experience. Pain is indeed a complex issue and may have to be looked at from a number of issues before it is resolved.

While counselling may benefit some people who are 'going round and round in circles' and appear unable to find their way through a problem, it isn't for everyone. The difficulty of being 'stuck' in a transitional state is that problems revolve round and round in a person's head and deepen the neurological pathway holding the memory. It then goes on default where the slightest thing triggers it off so the person is automatically drawn into remembering the traumatic event. Most of us will have the experience of the smell of baking taking us back to our childhood and standing in granny's kitchen. That memory has been captured and held in a neurological pathway for many decades.

Sometimes, problems cannot be all that easily solved. Not everyone will ever find out why they were singled out as the object of abuse when they were a child. Not everyone can forget the horrors of war. Talking about it does not always make it better sometimes the best response is to do as little to bring it to mind in the hope that the neurological pathway begins to fade and loses its default mechanism so that a stimulus triggers a different neurological memory with a different – hopefully happier – memory.

Fast and Slow Pain

A pain stimulus is transmitted through peripheral nerves to the spinal cord and from there to the brain. It can happen either through a fast nerve fibre or a slow one.

A fast pain is a sharp pain but after a few seconds this becomes a duller pain – like a burning pain. This can continue for days or weeks. Sometimes it can last much longer when it is classified as chronic pain.

Fast pain is transmitted by thick nerve fibres. They are called A-delta fibres. As they allow the pain stimulus to be transferred very quickly, it means that the body can react to a painful stimulus almost immediately and, as such, avoid any further damage.

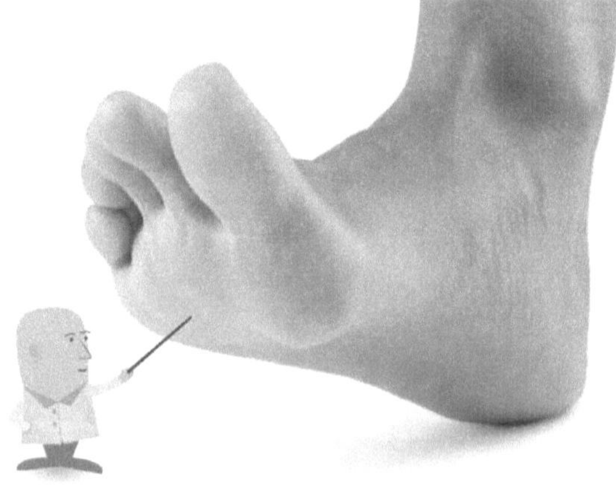

Fast pain is well localised. You will be able to locate the area of pain accurately as the pain is sharp.

Strong painkillers do not tend to work on this type of pain. This is why general or local anaesthetic is used in surgery since opioids will not take away the pain of a surgical incision.

Slow pain is transmitted by extremely thin nerve fibres known as C-nerve fibres. Their thin size means that pain can only be transmitted slowly to the brain.

Whereas a stimulus to fast fibres result in a quick response, a response to stimulus by slow nerve fibres results in immobilisation of the affected body part through guarding, holding it rigid or spasm. This allows healing to take place.

Slow pain is the primary type of pain which originates in internal organs. Localised trauma to the gut does not result in any pain.

However, when there is a much larger injury to internal organs such as when the bladder becomes distended because of a stone or even the pain of labour, the pain is poorly localised. The pain is diffuse and the origin cannot be firmly established by the patient. It may radiate, unlike fast pain. Gallstone pain can radiate from front to back. Kidney pain can be felt around the shoulder blade and the pain from a heart attack can be felt in the neck or the arm.

Opioids work very well on slow pain. Local anaesthetics block all nerve transmission and also work well on slow pain.

Characteristics of Fast and Slow pain

Slow pain	Fast Pain
Transmitted by thin nerves	**Transmitted by thicker nerves**
Poorly localised	**Well localised**
Felt in all internal organs except the brain	**Mainly felt in skin, anus and mouth**
Causes Immobilisation of injured part	**Immediate withdrawal of stimulation**
Pain may be referred	**Pain does not radiate**
Effective relief from opioids	**Little or no relief from opioids**
Pain from gallstones	**Pain from a cut**

Do fast and slow nerve fibres end in different parts of the brain?

The impulse from the slow pain is distributed diffusely in the brain and, as such, each area in the brain elicits a different response. This explains why slow pain can cause a wide range of symptoms such as

- Sleeplessness
- Mood changes
- Restlessness
- Loss of appetite

On the other hand the impulse from the fast nerve fibre travels to a very specific area on the surface of the brain in the cortex. This allows us to feel the precise localisation of the pain stimulus.

Why does Capsaicin block pain?

Pain receptors become exhausted very quickly if an ointment containing capsaicin is used. In a similar vein, a meal containing cayenne peppers or red and green chilli peppers is high in capsaicin and will also help to exhaust pain signals.

Substances released inside the body which contribute to pain.

Although we tend to think of chemical pain receptors being stimulated by chemicals in our environment, there are a good number of chemicals which originate in our body which are released in response to inflammation and trauma among other stimuli.

Redness and heat which occur at the site of injury are due to increased blood flow to the site of inflammation. The swelling is caused by an accumulation of fluid. This presses on nerve endings causing pain. Pain is also due to the release of substances that stimulate pain receptors or the lack of substances which would help ameliorate pain.

Some of these substances are
- Potassium ions
- Lactic acid
- Bradykinins
- Prostaglandins
- Histamine
- Serotonin
- Enkephalins

Pharmacological increase of peripheral potassium ion channel activity consistently alleviated pain in laboratory tests. This simply means that the more potassium ions were shunted down potassium channels in the cell walls the more that pain was likely to be alleviated. This action, of course, would depend on there being enough potassium in the diet in the first place. Potassium losses through the use of diuretics and/or laxatives could increase the potential for pain.

Prunes, dates, raisins, bananas and tomatoes are just some food items which are rich in potassium.

Lactic acid is the acid which causes muscle pain after heavy exercise. It builds up and irritates nerve endings. When our muscles are sore we rub them which stimulates different nerves not connected with transmitting pain from sore muscles.

Sometimes, sore muscles are a result of microscopic tears in muscle after heavy exercise.

Bradykinin is released in response to tissue injury is implicated in chronic pain. Some bradykinin inhibitors which suppress trauma-induced swelling are:-
- Bromelain
- Aloe
- Polyphenols found in red wine and green tea

When there are microscopic tears, ibuprofen and NSAIDS's should not be taken immediately, nor should warm baths. Both can cause bleeding from the microscopic tears, increasing pain. Athletes sit in baths of ice cold water after major exercise to reduce any pain and damage caused by these tiny tears. The same rule applies to sprains and strains which should be treated initially with cold compresses. After two or three days when any microscopic bleeding into the tissue is likely to have resolved then alternate hot and cold compresses will help healing substances flow to the site of injury and assist in removing toxic waste products.

When we encounter painful stimuli, chemicals called prostaglandins are released alongside them. They increase the sensitivity of pain receptors.

Non-steroidal anti-inflammatory drugs (NSAIDS) work well for this type of pain as they reduce the effect of prostaglandins. They act on the peripheral nervous system.

Paracetamol also works well on this type of pain but paracetamol operates from the central nervous system.
Sometimes, when you go to the GP, they will suggest that you take paracetamol and ibuprofen (NSAID) for pain. Taken this way their ability to reduce pain exceeds the ability of each separate painkiller if added together.

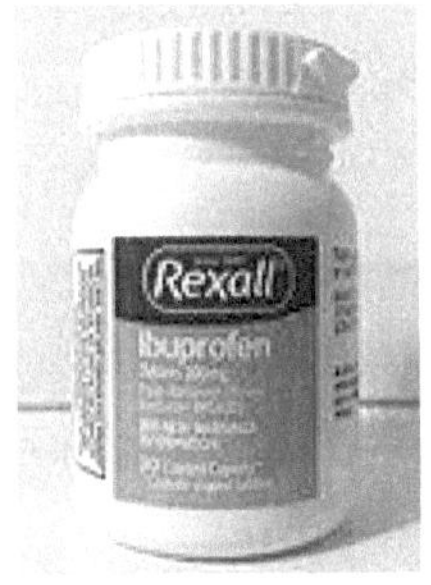

Ibuprofen reduces the effect of prostaglandins, reducing the sensitivity of pain receptors.

Antihistamines can also be useful in inhibiting pain. Most people associate antihistamines with allergic reactions such as hay fever and urticaria and have never considered them as useful drugs which can help to reduce pain levels.

Histamine is a vasoactive amine which has an important role in the early acute inflammatory response. It is stored in the granules of mast cells, basophils and platelets. Histamine is released from cells by stimuli which include acute inflammation. Histamine increases vasodilation - that is it widens blood vessels. It also makes them more permeable too. Histamine is a chemical mediator and brings immune system substances to the site of injury. The swelling and other substances irritate pain receptors causing pain.

Some patients cannot take NSAID's such as ibuprofen for various reasons. They may be hypersensitive to ibuprofen or be on medication such as methotrexate where such anti inflammatories are not recommended. In these cases an alternative painkiller should be sought to be taken alongside paracetamol. Some anti-histamines

Why do opioids work on pain?

The brain has a natural brake on pain. Once a pain stimulus hits the brain, the brain leaps into action and sends a signal back to the spinal cord to reduce the pain signal.

Two important molecules in this process are serotonin and encephalin.

Serotonin is a chemical which nerve cells produce which allows messages to be passed between nerve cells. It is mostly found in the digestive system but it can be found in blood platelets and serum, too.

The messages it passes along are related to mood, sexual desire, memory and learning, appetite, sleep and temperature regulation among others. Serotonin also has a major role to play in modulating pain perception. Serotonergic drugs are use in the treatment of migraine headaches.

In the spinal cord enkephalins inhibit painful sensations. They react with specific receptor sites on the sensory nerve endings. They bind to opiate receptors and release controlled amounts of pain so that we are not overwhelmed by them. Enkephalin is a natural opioid. Other natural opioids are endorphins and dynorphin.

Compounds such as enkephalins which inhibit pain are eventually degraded by enzymes which are called enkephalinases. If we can prevent the breakdown of enkephalins then painful sensations are inhibited for longer.

D-phenylalanine is an amino acid which inhibits encephalin degradation. Major dietary sources are meat, fish, eggs, cheese and milk. We shall look at D-phenylalanine in more detail, later.

The morphine administered in hospital wards works on the very same opioid receptors to block pain perception.

Why does being hungry shut off the perception of pain?

Studies have shown that avoiding pain is a necessary survival skill. Research has shown that a neural pathway was activated in mice who were hungry. This inhibited the perception of and response to chronic pain.

Fasting is often recommended as it has a number of health benefits. It may be that a new health benefit is its ability to reduce pain.

Why does rubbing the affected part suppress pain?

It is an instinctive reaction to rub an injured part of the body when it is hurt. There is a good reason why we do this. Rubbing or pressing stimulates other nerve fibres and they have first choice over the nerve fibres which are transmitting pain.

Herbal Supplements which are natural painkillers

- **Alpha lipoic acid**
- **Curcumin**
- **Fish oil**
- **Ginger**
- **Resveratrol**
- **spirulina**

These supplements are considered to be natural painkillers. We will examine the composition of them to see why.

Alpha lipoic acid
 Alpha-lipoic is an anti-oxidant and therefore has anti-inflammatory actions. Studies have shown that it has beneficial effects on back pain[3] although alpha-lipoic acid was also used in conjunction with gamma linoleic acid

---

[3] http://europepmc.org/abstract/med/19887043

Curcumin

Turmeric is that well known yellow spice which turns curry yellow. The active compound in turmeric is curcumin which has antioxidant and anti- inflammatory activity which helps promote healing. Studies have shown that it has pain-reducing abilities which can be as potent as over the counter medications. In clinical studies, curcumin's anti-inflammatory activity is beneficial for rheumatoid arthritis as well as a number of bowel disorders such as Crohn's disease, ulcerative colitis and irritable bowel syndrome.

There is only a small amount of curcumin in turmeric but capsules of curcumin are available at health food stores.

Ginger

Ginger has similar properties to curcumin in that it is antioxidant and anti-inflammatory in nature. Ginger is also able to help in cases of nausea which is an additional benefit over and above curcumin.

Fish Oil

Prostaglandins can either promote or reduce inflammation. Fish oils contain high concentrations of omega-3 fatty acids. These have been proven to shift the balance from the prostaglandins that increase inflammation to those that lessen it.

Spirulina
Spirulina is reputed to lessen the inflammatory response through anti-oxidative and anti-inflammatory mechanisms. It appears to break the cross talk between oxidative stress and inflammation.

The above are natural pain killers because they have anti-oxidative powers and are anti-inflammatory in action.

Free radicals, oxidative stress and inflammation

Free radicals are atoms or groups of atoms which have an unpaired electron. This can occur when oxygen interacts with certain molecules. These free radicals then behave a bit like an out of control pinball knocking into cells and DNA, damaging them in the process. As a result cells may die.

Some of the degenerative disorders which can result from free radicals are
- cataracts
- Alzheimer's disease
- Certain cancers
- Accelerated aging
- Some cancers
- Heart attacks
- Arthritis

Inflammation is part of the body's natural healing process but sometimes it becomes excessive and prolonged. When this happens problems will arise. Chronic inflammation is now known to be an underlying factor in most debilitating diseases.

A vicious cycle begins when free radical damage results in inflammation. Chronic inflammation produces lots of free radicals which go onto creating more inflammation. Chronic inflammation is like an out of control forest fire in your body.

Philip Schauer, MD, director of the Bariatric and Metabolic Institute at eh Cleveland Clinic stated, 'Chronic inflammation plays a direct role in diabetes, high blood pressure, sleep apnoea, asthma and other conditions.'

Antioxidants neutralise free radicals so that they can no longer cause damage and the subsequent inflammatory response. Antioxidants effectively put a brake on chronic inflammation and prevent the insidious and uncontrolled damage that is going on inside you.

There are many antioxidants. The three main vitamins with antioxidant activity are

- Vitamin A and its precursor beta-carotene. Vitamin A is fat soluble and is found in liver, cheese, butter and oily fish. Its precursor is found in collards and orange coloured vegetables such as carrot and pumpkin.

- Vitamin C – vitamin C is found in fresh fruit and vegetables. It is water soluble and is easily destroyed by cooking.
- Vitamin E – this is a fat soluble vitamin and is mainly found in nuts and wheat-germ.

Vitamin C and E work alongside each other in the brain. Vitamin E neutralises oxidants and vitamin C recycles any residue and activates it.

Vitamin E protects fatty acids in the brain, slows down neurodegeneration and the potential for microglia to develop and maintain chronic pain.

Lycopene is a bright red carotene found in tomatoes, papayas and watermelons which also has antioxidant properties.

Dark chocolate, red wine, spices such as cinnamon and nutmeg and yellow mustard seed all have antioxidant properties.

Redness and heat which occur at the site of injury are due to increased blood flow to the site of inflammation. The swelling is caused by an accumulation of fluid. This presses on nerve endings causing pain. Pain is also due to the release of chemicals such as bradykinin and histamine that stimulate pain receptors.

Magnesium as an analgesic

More and more the benefits of magnesium in relieving pain and inflammation are becoming known. Studies have found that at the cellular level, magnesium reduces inflammation. It was found that when an inflammatory condition is produced then a magnesium deficiency is created. Increasing magnesium intake decreases inflammation.

Magnesium is actively required by 700 enzyme systems in the body and there are a number of ways in which magnesium helps to reduce inflammation. Magnesium has been found to be a natural calcium channel blocker. This is important as excessive calcium is one of the most pro-inflammatory substances in the body.

The ratio of calcium to magnesium is held to be in the ratio of 800:400mg but more recent studies have argued that the amount of magnesium should equal that of calcium intake.

Dr Joseph Mercola DO has been quoted as saying

'We are all going to die at some point, but if you're deficient in magnesium you may wind up dying sooner rather than later.'

Research has shown that magnesium can be effective in both muscle and nerve pain. It is fairly clear that magnesium ameliorates muscles by its muscle relaxing abilities. It is these properties which are harnessed in the Epsom salt type bath crystals. However, a study on rats which appeared in the *Journal of Physiology* confirmed that magnesium decreases nerve pain.

N-methyl-D-aspartate (NMDA) is a pain carrying neurotransmitter. When this neurotransmitter is stimulated it is a major mechanism of pain. Some drugs such as Amantadine and Ketamine which help decrease and balance this neurotransmitter have significant side effects. For example, some of the side effects of Amantadine are listed as being

- Depression, anxiety and irritability
- Hallucinations and confusion
- Anorexia
- Dry mouth
- Constipation
- Somnolence
- agitation

among many others.

However, magnesium has been found to calm down NMDA without the side effects that most of the prescription drugs have.

The authors of the above study have argued that magnesium deficiency can be a major amplifier of pain and have highlighted that most people are magnesium deficient.

The only contraindication to supplementing with magnesium is for those who have kidney disease

Magnesium supplementation for migraine

Magnesium oxide is often used to prevent migraine at a dose of 500mg daily. Evidence for magnesium's effectiveness is in patients who have had aura with their migraines where it is thought that magnesium may prevent waves of brain signalling. These waves –cortical spreading depression – initiate the visual and sensory changes associated with aura.

Magnesium also decreases the release of substance P and glutamate as well as preventing the narrowing of brain blood vessels caused by the neurotransmitter serotonin.

Substance P and glutamate are pain transmitting chemicals.
Substance P is released from the ends of specific sensory nerves and is found in the central and peripheral nervous system. It is associated with inflammatory processes and pain.

Neuronal substance P is stored in vesicles and released when it comes into contact with
- leukotrienes
- prostaglandins
- histamine

among others

Ginger blocks both the production of prostaglandins and leukotrienes. In cell based studies capsaicin (found in peppers) and curcumin both blocked the production of leukotrienes.

Ibuprofen blocks prostaglandins.

Antihistamines block histamine release.

The inflammatory processes of Substance P and the subsequent pain can be addressed by over the counter medications.

Glutamate is a neurotransmitter which is associated with pain transmission. It is neurotoxic and has to be kept inside neurons. It's concentration in cells is much larger than the small amount released at crucial times.   A healthy neuron only releases glutamate when it needs to pass on a message. If too much is released pumps in the membrane suck the excess back.
When damaged cells release their glutamate the neuron isn't killed directly. The cell is excited and its pores are opened too much this allows excessive quantities of salt and calcium into the cell.

Sodium causes cell swelling which presses on adjacent blood vessels. This can ultimately lead to cell death and the release of further glutamate from damaged cells. However, this is reversible if glutamate is removed from brain fluids.

Calcium is more of a thug. If it rushes through open pores excessively it destroys the neuron's vital structures and eventually kills it. Dead cells will continue to spew out glutamate destroying areas of brain until the glutamate pumps are able to overcome the extra cellular glutamate and return it to the safety of the cell.

Alpha-Lipoic Acid – found in spinach, broccoli and liver helps glutamate transport proteins which help remove excess extracellular glutamate. [4]

The flavonoid agipenin which is found in parsley, celery, thyme, cloves, lemon balm and chamomile, among others inhibits glutamate. In culture it was found to be neuroprotective against glutamate-induced neurotoxicity in cerebellar and corticol neurons[5]. An antagonistic effect of apigenin on GABA and NMDA was found.

GABA is a neurotransmitter which has calming and pain relieving properties. Rosmarinic acid, which is found in oregano, lemon balm, sage, marjoram and rosemary, increases GABA levels by inhibiting an enzyme which converts GABA to L-glutamate.

---

[4] http://www.jpands.org/vol9no2/blaylock.pdf
[5] https://www.ncbi.nlm.nih.gov/pubmed/15464088

The olive leaf contains oleuropein which prevents against damage from bacteria and insects. It helps to relieve intestinal spasms so is useful for pain from irritable bowel syndrome.

 Studies show that oleuropein dissolves the outer lining of micro-organisms thus destroying them. It is also an antioxidant and therefore has anti-inflammatory properties. It has been shown to inhibit cancerous cells in the breast, bladder and brain.

A study published in the Pakistan Journal of Biological Sciences found that a salve made of ginger, cinnamon and sesame oil was just as effective as the over counter medication creams containing salicylate which is a topical analgesic

Amino acids, antioxidant, anti-inflammatory and pain relieving properties.

Amino acids are the building blocks of protein and, as such are found in all animal foods Peas, beans and other legumes are rich sources of animal protein.

Amino acids can be non–essential, that is they can be made in the body, or essential which means they must be taken in through diet. Some amino acids are also said to be conditional which means that normally the body can make them but at times of illness or injury, they may need to be ingested or supplemented.

Methionine, cartilage and arthritis.

Professor and Dr Klaus Miehlke was classed as the leading expert on bone diseases in Germany. He has argued that in cases of joint or cartilage disease, it is of the utmost importance that the human body receives the cartilage-forming substances in sufficient quantities. He states that a healthy diet cannot provide this and recommends supplements which contain cartilage-forming substances.

Methionine is one such cartilage forming substance. It is an essential amino acid which means it must be taken in from the diet.

Methionine donates sulphur and joint cartilage requires sulphur for its creation. Tests have shown that cartilage in healthy individuals contains around three times more sulphur than in patients who suffer from arthritis.   Patients who have arthritis are advised to supplement with methionine and the B vitamins to optimise the results.

Methionine has particular importance in three main areas

- it stimulates the cartilage cells to create more cartilaginous tissue

- contains anti- inflammatory properties

- has an analgesic effect

Dietary sources of methionine include onions, garlic, eggs, meat, fish, sesame seeds, nuts. Most fruit and vegetables contain little methionine although sulphur containing compounds are found in Brussels sprouts and broccoli.

Arginine helps create new bone therefore it is particularly useful for those with a propensity towards osteoporosis.

Arginine supports the production of collagen which is a protein which is a basic component of connective tissues like cartilage. It also supports the growth of osteoblasts which are cells which form new bone.

When a deficiency of arginine occurs it can cause osteoporosis. Studies have shown that arginine in combination with other amino acids supported the growth of osteoblasts[6] It was therefore recommended that the administration of amino acids belonged to all osteoporosis treatments.

---

[6] Ursini, F. & Pipicelli, G. (2009) *Nutritional Supplementation for Osteoarthritis,* Alternative and Complementary Therapies, Volume 15, issue 4, (pp. 173-177)

Arginine is found in all animal foods, soybeans, peanuts, walnuts and pumpkin seeds.

DL Phenylalanine – this essential amino acid has been well researched and documented and is effective in the control of chronic and acute pain syndromes which include

- lower back pain

- osteoarthritis

- joint pain resulting from rheumatoid arthritis

- migraine

- neuralgia

among others

DLPA appears to focus on chronic pain only. It protects the brain own natural endorphins allowing them to continue to act effectively and for longer periods than that of pharmaceutical products.

DLPA has also been found to have strong antidepressant action and is effective in relieving anxiety.

Good sources of phenylalanine are animal foods and beans and nuts. During illness when appetite is lost and phenylalanine levels are also below optimum levels then pain is likely to increase. Phenylalanine supplementation should be considered at this time and is available in powdered form and is obtainable for health food shops or online.

Dosage initial dosage would be 2000mg increasing to no more than 4,500mg by two weeks. It is a good adjunctive therapy but can also be used alone.

Amino acids should always be taken on an empty stomach to maximise absorption. In free form they need no digesting and so can act within minutes – far quicker than prescribed medications unless they are the injectable form.

Glutamine is found in muscles. It is known as brain fuel as it easily passes through the blood brain barrier. Glutamine increases the amount of GABA – another amino acid and neurotransmitter - which inhibits pain. It is the amino acid found in the intestinal gut lining and helps conditions such as Crohn's disease, leaky gut syndrome and irritable bowel syndrome. Thus it helps address gut related pain and any damage caused by NSAID's such as ibuprofen.

The body's two primary pain modulators

The body has its own analgesic system which are the neurotransmitters. The two main ones are derived from amino acids

- Gamma amino butyric acid (GABA)

- Endorphins

It is perhaps no surprise that one of these precursor amino acids is DL phenylalanine. Seymour Ehrenpreis PhD., pharmacology professor at Chicago Medical School demonstrated that this endorphinase[7] allowed the medical school to significantly reduce the amounts of opiate medication administered.

Phenylalanine is also useful in reducing food cravings and can assist in weight loss.

---

[7] inhibits the breakdown of pain reliving endorphins

GABA

GABA is a major inhibitory neurotransmitter and helps calm pain and relieve anxiety. It is also an amino acid in its own right. For a long time GABA was not thought capable of crossing the blood brain barrier but more recently evidence has been found for the presence of a GABA transporter in the blood brain barrier. This demonstrates that GABA can enter or exit the brain.

A lack of inhibition by neurotransmitters – mainly GABA – is responsible for many pain states. Some GABA analogues such as Gabapentin and Pregabalin act by inhibiting ion channels which contributes to their analgesic effects.

Final Thoughts

When the root cause of pain and the different types of pain are understood then, this in itself, has the power to reduce levels of pain since it imbues a sense of power over something that once had control.

Pain is useful in telling us that something is wrong. Once that feat has been accomplished and we are able to address, as far as possible, the injury or illness contributing to the pain, then such discomfort is not really required.

Pain is debilitating and can reduce quality of life yet we do have our own pain relieving mechanisms in our bodies which sometimes just need a change in diet to be able to harness them.

I hope that this book helps in the understanding of pain in order that you know the best way to deal with it and, in doing so, can improve the quality of your life.